COMPUTER-INTEGRATED SURGERY